How to Stop Snoring Naturally

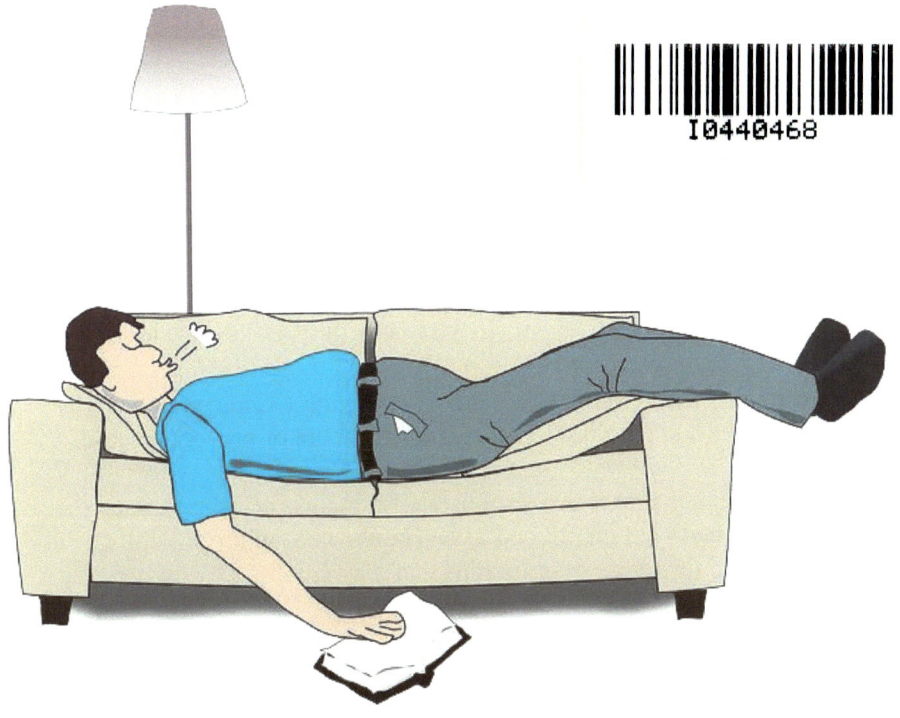

I0440468

M. Usman

Healthy Living Series

Mendon Cottage Books

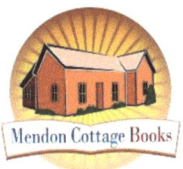

JD-Biz Publishing

Our books are available at

1. Amazon.com

2. Barnes and Noble

3. Itunes

4. Kobo

5. Smashwords

6. Google Play Books

Table of Contents

Preface

Around 45% of normal adults snore occasionally and around 25% are routine snorers. Though it may seem to be a normal problem, as it is very common, but it should not be taken carelessly, especially in case of habitual snorers, as it may be an indication of obstructed breathing.

Now a days, there are many anti- snoring devices available in the market and every year more of them are added, promising to cure the snoring problem. Unfortunately, many of these devices are not backed by research or lab testing. Some of them may even require you to stay awake the whole night.

However, there are plenty of proven techniques and natural remedies that can help in eliminating this problem instead of relying on these devices. In this eBook, we discuss snoring, sleeping disorders, what causes snoring, and natural remedies including home remedies to treat snoring. Apart from that, we also talk about how to deal with the snoring complaints and how to cooperate and ask your partner to support you in curing the problem.

Snoring

Chapter # 1: Snoring and its characteristics

Snoring is a loud noise that occurs while sleeping when air is not able to move freely through the nose and the throat; thus causing the surrounding tissues to vibrate and producing the sound.

People who snore may have excess of throat and nasal tissue, which is more prone to vibrate. Sometimes the position of the tongue may also obstruct the smooth breathing pattern.

Characteristics of Snoring:

- Though snoring can affect anyone, but it is more commonly seen in men and people who are overweight.

- Snoring worsens with age.

- The snoring sound may come either from nose, mouth or both and may occur during any time of sleep.

- It may cause a dry mouth or irritated throat after you wake up.

- Light snoring is considered normal and may not disrupt your overall sleep quality but heavy snoring may require medical attention.

There can be various reasons for snoring from congestion due to cold or allergies to consumption of alcohol or depressants which make your throat muscles relax.

In most of the cases people do not realize that they snore but more than half of people snore at some point in their lives.

Chapter # 2: Health risks associated with snoring

Snoring at some point in your lives or being an irregular snorer seems to be normal but habitual snorers may be at a risk of various health problems like heart disease, stroke, diabetes, and even sleep apnea (sleeping disorder).

Though snoring is a symptom of sleep apnea but not everyone who snores suffers from this disorder. Obstructive sleep apnea is a serious sleep disorder that causes you to stop breathing temporarily while sleeping.

Sleep apnea creates several other problems like:

- **Temporary interruption of breathing:** This may last from few seconds to minutes during sleep. It is caused by partial or total blockage of the airway.

- **Light Sleep or frequent waking from sleep:** Even though a sleeping person may not realize it but sleep apnea may cause frequent waking up from sleep. This interferes with normal sleeping pattern causing light sleep rather than deep and restorative sleep.

- **Health problems:** Prolonged sleep apnea results in poor night sleep leading to drowsiness during the day thus interfering with the quality of life. It may also result in high blood pressure with high risk of heart attack.

Remember, even after having sufficient sleep, if you feel tired all the time and your snoring is usually paired with choking, you may have sleep apnea. It's better to contact a medical expert who is trained to detect and diagnose this sleep disorder.

Causes of Snoring

Chapter # 3: Causes of Snoring

When the air flow between the nose and the mouth is obstructed, it results in snoring. This obstruction in the airflow can be due to various factors, including:

- **Infection or Allergies:** Some people snore during a sinus infection or during allergy season.

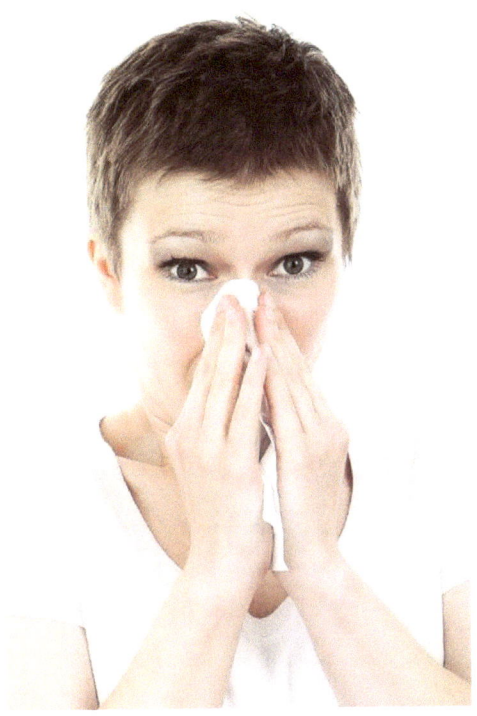

- **Deformity of the nose:** In case of any deformity of the nose such as a structural change in the wall separating one nostril from the other may also cause an obstruction resulting in snoring.

- **Poor toning of throat and tongue muscles:** Sometimes the throat and the tongue muscles can be too loose or relaxed, resulting into an obstruction in the airway. This could be also due to alcohol consumption, deep sleep, use of sleeping pills, or aging. These relaxed muscles may collapse and fall back in the airway.

- **Tonsils or bulky throat tissues:** Children with large tonsils often snore. Also, being overweight can cause throat tissues to become bulky and obstruct the normal airway. Even if one is not bulky but carrying excess weight around neck or throat may also result in snoring.

- **Age:** The normal aging process makes your throat become narrower and decreases the overall muscle tone of your throat, causing you to snore.

- **Long soft palate or uvula:** A long uvula (the dangling tissue in the back of the mouth) or a long soft palate may narrow the opening from nose to throat, causing vibration and obstruction in the airway thus resulting in snoring.

- **Gender:** Men tend to snore more than women, due to the fact that they have narrower air passages.

- **Heredity:** A narrow throat, a long palate, and other physical attributes that cause snoring may be hereditary.

- **Nasal Problems:** A plugged nose makes breathing in difficult and results in an emptiness in the throat, thus leading to snoring.

- **Smoking, Alcohol consumption, and medications:** Smoking, alcohol consumption, and use of certain medicines like tranquilizers can increase muscle relaxation and cause more snoring.

- **Sleep position:** Sleeping on back usually causes the throat muscles to relax and obstruct the airway.

Different people snore for different reasons. It's best to analyze why you snore and the root cause. Once you are able to find that, it will be very easy to work towards getting a deep, quiet sleep.

To do this, try maintaining a sleep diary with the help of your partner, to monitor your snoring patterns. This will help in knowing the reasons of your snoring, what makes it worse, and what steps need to be taken to stop it. These reasons may differ from behavioral or lifestyle factors to physical anatomy.

Remember, the main cause of snoring is the relaxation of mouth, nose, or throat muscles during sleep. When you move from light sleep to deep sleep, your muscles tend to relax and collapse back into the throat, thus narrowing the airway. Narrower the air passage becomes, more is the obstruction while breathing and more is the vibration which results into more loud and harsh snoring sound.

So it is important to know the cause of snoring before looking for a remedy as some solutions may alleviate the muscles to relax more instead of preventing them from obstructing the airway.

Chapter # 4: How you snore shows why you snore

There are certain indicators in the way you sleep and snore which give a high level cause of why you snore.

- **Closed mouth snoring:** If you snore with a closed mouth, your tongue maybe the problem.

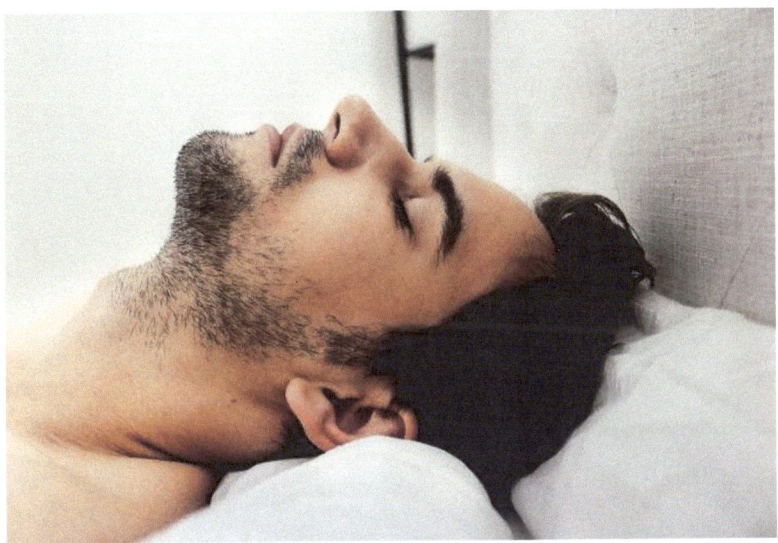

- **Open mouth snoring:** If you snore with an open mouth, it is related to the tissues in your throat.

- **Snoring while lying on your back:** Snoring when sleeping on your back is usually mild snoring. A little bit of lifestyle changes and improved sleep habits may cure it.

- **Snoring in all sleep positions:** Snoring while sleeping in any sleep position, may require proper treatment

Natural remedies to stop snoring

Chapter # 5: Tips to stop snoring naturally

Be it losing weight or changing your sleep position, the following are some of the tips and tricks which you can try to cure your snoring without taking any medicines:

- **Keep your head elevated:** Put some extra pillows under your head rather than lying flat on your back. This will prevent the tissues in the throat from falling in the air passages.

- **Elevate the bed:** Elevate the bed side where you keep your head while sleeping, by either placing several flat boards under the legs of the bed or opting for a bed which has a manual/automatic facility of raising its one side.

- **Sleep on one side:** Though it may sound like a difficult task and also there will be no guarantee that you will remain in the same position throughout the night, but try to start sleeping on your side. You may even wrap your arms around your pillow. Sleeping on your side rather than your back will restrict your tongue and soft palate from falling back or resting against your throat, thus keeping the airway clear of any blockages.

- **Ball at the back:** Try sewing in a little pouch at the back of your pajama top and tuck a ball inside it (example, a tennis ball). So whenever at night, if you'll roll on your back while sleeping, you'll get a nudge from the tennis ball, making you go back to your side again.

- **Decongestant:** If your snoring is being caused by nasal congestion, take a decongestant to improve inhalation before hitting your bed since a stuffed nose can make breathing difficult, especially at night. Neti-pots are yet another over the counter saline spray which clears nasal passages.

- **Nasal strips:** These are available at most drugstores. You can put one strip on the outside of your nose before you go to sleep. This will help in opening your nostrils and increasing the airflow.

- **Reduce allergens in the bedroom:** Allergens like dust, pet dander, etc increase the nasal stuffiness. Try to vacuum drapes and curtains, cleaning the floors, and changing the bed sheets and pillow covers often. Also try keeping pets outside the bedroom.

- **Use a peppermint mouthwash:** Gargling with a peppermint mouthwash will shrink the lining of your nose and throat. This is usually effective if your snoring is caused by a head cold or an allergy and is temporary. You can even gargle by mixing one drop of peppermint oil into a glass of cold water. Remember to only gargle and **do not** swallow it.

- **Use a neck brace:** You may also use a neck brace to stop your snoring. It helps in keeping your chin extended so that your throat doesn't bend and keeps your airway clear and open. There are various types of neck braces available in drug stores these days. Opt for a soft foam one, which is less restraining and will work just right for your snoring problem.

- **Lose weight:** Try losing some weight. This may help in easing down any restriction on your upper airway. Moderately working out a few days a week not only helps in curing your snoring but also helps in maintaining a consistent sleep schedule which is a suggested habit to stop snoring.

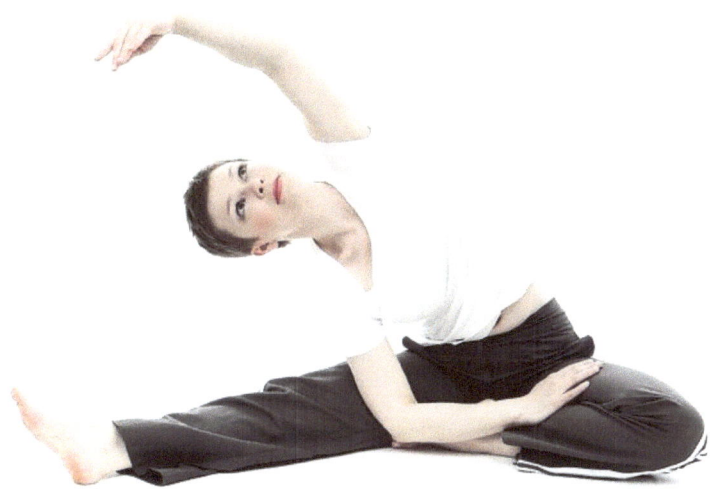

- **Drink herbal tea:** Some people are allergic to pollen that results into seasonal snoring problem. It is recommended that they drink tea made from the herb 'stinging nettle' just before their bedtime. This soothes the inflammation caused by the pollen allergens. To make this tea, pour one cup of boiling water over one tablespoon of the dried leaf. Cover the tea and keep it aside for 5-7 minutes. Strain it and drink. These herbal leaves are available in health food stores.

- **Avoid a heavy meal:** Try to avoid taking in a heavy meal or snack before two hours of your bedtime as it may cause your throat muscles to relax.

- **Quit smoking:** Tobacco smoke irritates the mucous membranes and may cause upper airway inflammation and irritation. The throat may swell, leading to narrowing of the airway. Regular smokers may have a problem with nasal congestion and prolonged smoking may lead to permanent damage to the respiratory system.

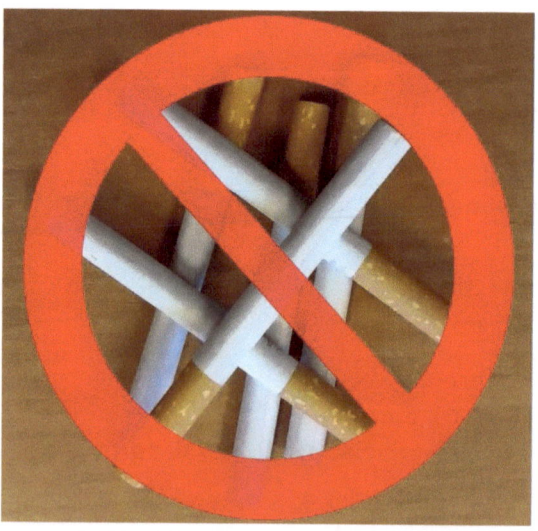

- **Avoid alcohol or any alcoholic beverages:** Try to avoid having any alcoholic beverages within three hours of your bedtime as it will make your throat muscles relax more than normal.

- **Use a humidifier:** Dry air may also cause snoring. You may use a good humidifier in your bedroom which will keep your air passage moist. Remember to clean it regularly. Another approach to fight with dry air could be using a steam vaporizer i.e. just before bedtime, take a bowl of hot water, bend over the bowl while draping a towel over your head. Your nose should be roughly 15-20 centimeters away from the bowl. Breathe deeply through your nose for a few minutes.

- **Check on your medicines:** If you are regularly taking any medication, you may want to opt for an alternative by consulting your doctor. There are some drugs which may make snoring worse like sleeping pills or other sedatives.

- **Establish a sleep routine:** Having a good night sleep is one of the natural ways to stop snoring. Going to bed and getting up at the same time creates a biological sleep-wake cycle. This helps ensure that your body gets plenty of quality sleep. When we are tired, we usually experience deep sleep that relaxes our throat airway more than normal, similar to drinking alcohol or taking a sedative, thus resulting in snoring.

Chapter # 6: Bedtime remedies

It's important to follow certain bedtime routines as a remedy to cure snoring like:

- **Keep bedroom air moist:** If swollen tissues are a problem, it could be due to dry air. In such cases a humidifier may help.

- **Use saline:** In case of a plugged nose, rinse your sinuses with a saline solution before going to bed. Neti pots, nasal decongestants, or nasal strips maybe useful.

- **Use an anti-snoring mouth appliance:** These are similar to an athlete's mouth guard and help in opening your airway by bringing your lower jaw and tongue forward during sleep. A DIY (do-it-yourself) kit will always be cheaper than the dentist made appliance. Apart from nasal strips, there are nasal dilators which are placed inside the nose to push the nostrils apart for easy airflow. Chin strips are also available which can be taped under your chin, thus helping stop the mouth from opening during sleep.

- **Quality Sleep:** Get quality sleep by sticking to a bed time routine. Try elevating your head side of the bed for easy breathing. You can either use a couple of soft pillows (there are specially designed pillows available to help in preventing snoring that ensure that your neck muscles are not strained) or elevate the head side of your bed by putting few blocks under the legs of your bed. And moreover try sleeping on your sides rather than back.

- **Avoid foods and beverages that relax your throat muscles:** Try to avoid foods and beverages like alcohol before bedtime, which may relax your throat muscles more than normal.

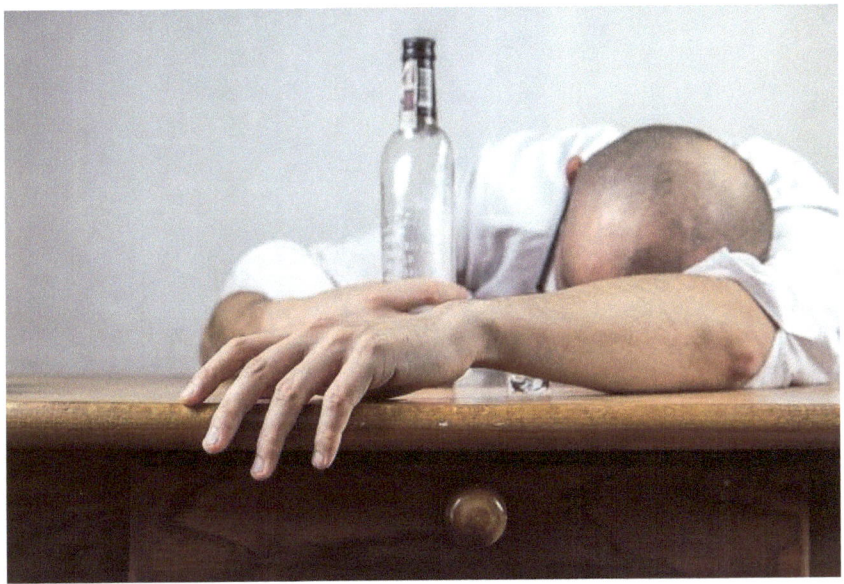

- **Avoid exercising too close to bedtime:** Exercising too close to bedtime may keep you awake longer.

Chapter # 7: Throat exercises

Throat exercises when practiced daily, help in strengthening the muscles of your the upper breathing tract and can be an effective way to reduce snoring problems.

If you have a busy schedule and are not able to find time to practice these exercises, there are some exercises, which can be performed while doing your housework, while taking a shower, or walking your dog.

It's advisable (just as with any workout routine) to start slow and gradually increase the number of reps in a set.

Following are some of the effective throat exercises:

- Place the tip of your tongue behind your top front teeth. Now slide the tongue backwards for three minutes a day. You can do it for three minutes at a stretch or for one minute each three times a day.

- With an open mouth, move your jaw to one side and hold for 30 seconds and then repeat the same thing on the other side.

- Repeat each vowel (a-e-i-o-u) out loud for three minutes, a few times a day.

- With an open mouth, contract the muscles in the back of your throat repeatedly for 30 seconds. You may look in the mirror to see the hanging ball (uvula) in your mouth moving up and down.

- Close your mouth and press your lips and hold for 30 seconds. Repeat 5 times.

Alternate exercises:

- **Singing:** Singing helps in increasing the muscle tone and control of the throat and the soft palate thus reducing the snoring.

- **Playing any wind instrument:** Research shows that learning a wind instrument like didgeridoo can help in strengthening the throat and soft palate muscles thus reducing snoring.

Chapter # 8: Home remedies for curing snoring

There are various products and devices available in market today to treat snoring. Each product has its own degree of pros and cons. Some products may prove to be not as effective as they claim to be.

Though there is no magic to cure snoring but certain lifestyle changes and some simple home remedies may help in controlling it to a great extent.

The following are some of the home remedies which must be given a try before opting for any medication:

- **Olive Oil:**

   Olive oil is a strong anti-inflammatory and eases the tissues of the respiratory passage, thus reducing the swelling and soreness and keeping the air passage clear of any obstruction. Regular use of olive oil also lessens the vibrations in the throat and can cure snoring completely.

   How to apply:

   o   Mix half teaspoon of olive oil with equal amount of honey. Consume it daily before bed.

   OR

   o   Consume two or three sips of olive oil daily before going to bed.

- **Clarified Butter:**

  Also known as 'ghee', has medicinal value that helps in opening up the nasal passages and softening the tissues of the respiratory glands, thus helping in snoring less and sleeping better.

  How to apply:

  o Warm a small amount of clarified butter in microwave or on gas burner. With the help of a dropper, put two to three drops of lukewarm clarified butter in each nostril. Do it daily before hitting the bed and after waking up the next morning.

- **Peppermint:**

  Peppermint is yet another anti inflammatory ingredient that helps in reducing the swelling of the membranes in the lining of the throat and the nostrils. This eases the breathing.

  Peppermint works very well in case of snoring caused due to allergy, cold, and dry air i.e. wherein the snoring problem is temporary.

  How to apply:

  o Gargle with peppermint oil water (One or two drops of peppermint oil to an 8 ounce glass of water) before going to bed. Ensure that you **don't swallow it**. Repeat this daily until you get the desired results.

    OR

- Add a few drops of peppermint oil to a humidifier about 30 minutes before going to bed. Run the humidifier overnight. This will help in opening your blocked airways and help in restricting snoring.

  OR

- Rub a little peppermint oil onto the lower portions of your nose before going to bed.

- **Cardamom:**

  Cardamom is an excellent expectorant and decongestant, making it effective for opening up blocked nasal passages, thus resulting in less snoring.

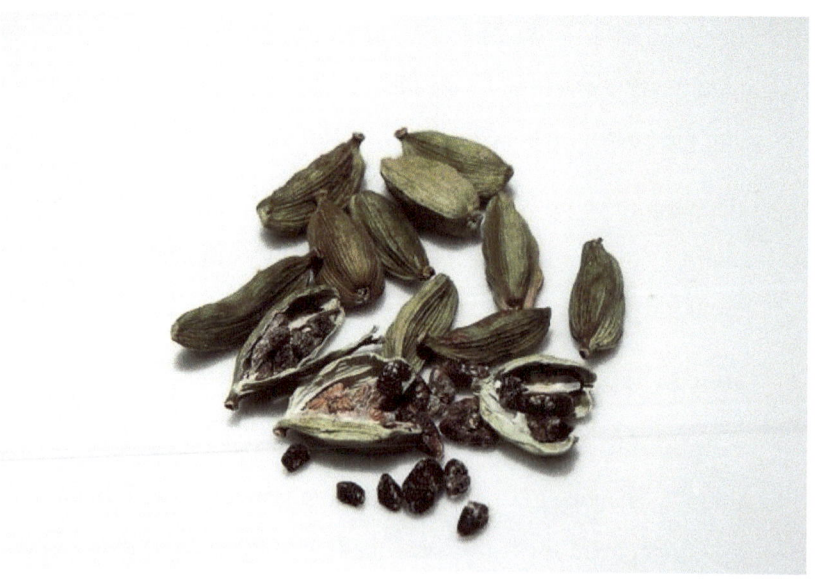

How to apply:

o   Add one half teaspoon of cardamom powder to a glass of warm water and drink it daily 30 minutes before going to bed. Doing it regularly will gradually reduce the snoring.

- **Steam:**

Inhaling steam is the best solution for reducing nasal congestion which is the main reason behind snoring.

How to apply:

o   Take hot boiling water in a large bowl. Add three to four drops of tea tree oil or eucalyptus oil in it. Take a towel and cover your head and inhale the steam deeply through your nose for around 10 minutes. You may repeat it daily before going to bed until your congestion clears.

- **Turmeric:**

Turmeric is a powerful antiseptic and antibiotic. It helps in treating inflammation and thus reducing heavy snoring. It should be consumed with milk. Turmeric not only helps in treating snoring and making you breathe freely but it also gives a boost to your immune system.

How to apply:

o   Add two teaspoons of turmeric to 8 ounces of warm milk. Drink it at least half an hour before going to sleep. Avoid consuming any other liquid after that. Do this daily.

Dealing with your snoring complaints

Chapter # 9: Communicating with your partner

No matter how much you love and care for your loved ones, snoring can put a strain on your relationship. If you are the snorer, you are bound to feel helpless, guilty or may even get irritated by your partner's complaining about something you cannot control. If you are the partner who lies awake the whole night, it's obvious very soon your aggression and irritation will take a toll on you and your partner.

Relationship problems do crop up if one partner snores and apart from resulting into communication breakdown whenever the problem is discussed, it may also result into:

- **Sleep deprivation:** Sleep loss or disturbed sleep may lead to irritability. Not only is the partner of the snorer, but the snorer himself/herself is unable to sleep properly because of the disordered breathing. Poor sleep thus takes a toll on the thinking skills and mood and may result into irritability, stress and conflicts.

- **Sleeping in separate rooms:** Though this may seem to be the easy way around the problem for couples, it does take a toll on your physical, as well as your emotional intimacy. If you are the snorer, you are bound to feel lonely or punished for something which is out of your control.

- **Partner resentment:** It happens when the non-snorer partner feels that he/she has done everything to sleep through the night (for example, use of ear plugs, sound machines, etc) but the snorer is not taking any effort to combat his/her snoring, it may lead to a feeling of resentment.

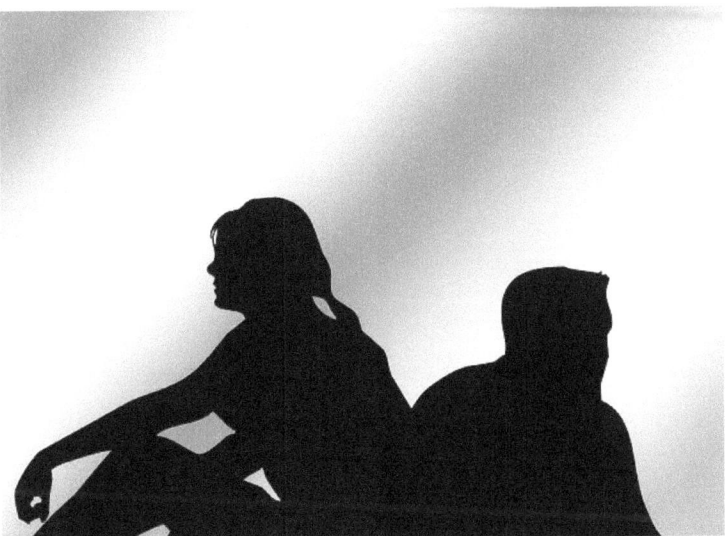

- So if you value your relationship, it's important to work as a team and find a cure of the snoring problem which not only will prevent future disagreements but will also help both of you to sleep soundly.

- It may even help in improving the quality of the bond you share and stay deeply connected to each other.

The following are some of the tips to help you to tackle the issue sensitively and maturely:

- **Be concerned:** It's pretty normal to get impatient and irritated about your partner's snoring habits. Even the most patient person is bound to draw the line at sleep loss. But remember, no matter how much sleep you lose due to your partner's snoring, try to handle the problem sensitively. Try to park your frustration on the problem rather than the person. No doubt, your partner feels equally defensive, helpless, and even embarrassed about his/her snoring problem.

- **Beware of getting rude:** Ensure that discussing the issue is not an outlet of your hidden frustrations. No doubt, sleep deprivation may have been damaging to your health, but try to approach the issue in a more resolution and helpful mode.

- **Right time to discuss:** Avoid discussing the issue when you are feeling exhausted like the middle of the night or early morning.

- **Use your playfulness:** Keep in mind that your partner is not keeping you awake on purpose. So try to bring up the subject without hurting your partner's feelings but do not overdo it. Laughing it out, imitating the sound may just ease the tension.

Chapter # 10: Dealing with the snoring complaints

It is obvious to feel hurt or embarrassed when your partner complains about your snoring habit. After all, it is purely unintentional and you probably didn't realize it was happening.

Though it might seem strange that snoring can cause havoc in a relationship, it's a very common and real problem. So whenever your partner complains about your snoring problem, try not to ignore it, and refuse to try solving the issue. This will very clearly send a message of 'unconcerned' about your partner's needs.

Take the matter seriously and try looking out for a solution with your partner. Also, keep following things in mind as you and your partner work together to find a solution to your snoring problem:

- **Do not take it personally:** Try not to take the complaints too personally. Your partner's frustrations are not for you but for your snoring.

- **Take your partner seriously:** Be patient and listen to your partner seriously. Remember, sleep loss is a health hazard which may make your partner feel miserable for rest of the day.

- **Ask for help and be cooperative:** Do not shy away from asking for help of your partner in solving the problem and try to be cooperative.

- **Snoring is a physical issue:** Remember it's just a physical issue and you are not alone, 6 out of 10 people snore. There is nothing to be embarrassed about. It could just be due to common cold or a relaxed muscle, improving on which is in your hands.

- **Give priority to your relationship:** If you and your partner understand the issue, it would be easy for both of you to cure the issue without losing each other.

- **Give a solution:** You understand that sleep deprivation may lead to moodiness and irritability. Let your partner know that it's okay to wake you up, if you start snoring at night rather than poking or shouting.

Chapter # 11: Self defense

It could be your partner, your room mate, or any of your family or friends who are facing the issue of snoring. Remember, there is nothing like 'God help me' frustration. There are many who have dealt with the issue and have resolved it with patience rather than spoiling their relationships. So before you start losing out, try opting for some methods which may lessen your frustrations for your otherwise lovable bedmate.

Following are some of the self defense methods which you can apply:

- **Buy a pair of earplugs:** Earplugs are quite comfortable, once you get accustomed to it and are inexpensive too.

- **Sleep early:** Try to hit the bed earlier than your partner so that at least you have a sound start on a good night sleep.

- **Go for an electronic noise machine:** There are various electronic machines available in the market that soften the outside noise and make your bedroom calmer. Opting for this type of a device, may make the night with the snorer more bearable.

Chapter #12: When to see a doctor

Though snoring seems to be a natural and physical issue, but it may be a warning sign of a serious problem. Loud, excessive snoring may signal sleep apnea (a dangerous condition which may require immediate treatment).

A doctor or a specialist should be able to evaluate a snorer for any of the sleep related breathing problems or sleeping disorders.

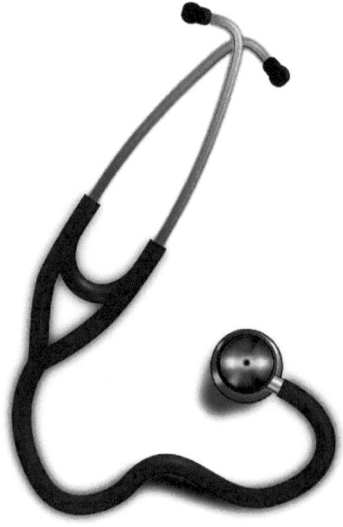

It's important to call your doctor if you or your sleep partner notices any of the following things:

- You snore loudly and harshly and are usually tired during the day even after sleeping for sufficient hours.

- You choke, gasp or even stop breathing during sleep.

- You wake up with a headache.

- You fall sleep at inappropriate times like during a meal, a conversation, or even while driving.

Sleep apnea may reduce levels of oxygen in the blood resulting into high levels of blood pressure and an inflated or puffy heart. To rule out the seriousness of the problem, the doctor may refer you to a sleep specialist for doing certain home based sleep test using a portable monitor and devices such as a continuous positive airway pressure (CPAP) or may even request you to stay overnight at a sleep clinic.

If the sleep studies and test conclude that your snoring is not related to any of the sleeping or breathing disorders, you may discuss other treatment options like lifestyle modifications (changing sleep position, losing weight, physical changes of the bed or the pillows, etc) to cure the snoring problem.

If the sleep tests show any underlying sleep or breathing problem, remember there is nothing to be panicked about. Surgeries are possible for the same. Your ENT doctor or physician may recommend a medical device or surgical procedure such as:

- **Traditional surgery:** It usually increases the size of your airway by surgically correcting the abnormalities or clearing the hindering tissues.

- **Laser assisted Uvulopalatoplasty (LAUP):** It uses lasers to shorten the uvula and to make small cuts on the either side of the soft palate. As these cuts heal, the surrounding tissues stiffen to prevent vibrations that result into snoring.

- **Continuous Positive Airway Pressure (CPAP):** It's a machine that blows pressurized air into your mask that is to be put on the nose throughout the night. Kept near your bedside, it helps in keeping your airway open during the night.

- **Implants:** Also known as the pillar procedure. The procedure involves inserting small plastic implants inside the soft palate, thus preventing the collapse of the soft palate which may be the cause of snoring.

- **Somnoplasty:** It is a small surgical operation of say around 30 minutes which uses low levels of radiofrequency heat to remove excessive tissues of the soft palate and the uvula which vibrate while snoring and create the sound.

Conclusion

Though there are many natural remedies which can help in curing your snoring problem. But do remember that not every remedy is right for every person. It may require a lot of patience, experiment, willingness to try different solutions, lifestyle changes, etc to come out with a solution and remedy that works for you.

References

http://www.sleepeducation.com

http://www.medicinenet.com

http://www.medicinenet.com/snoring/article.htm

About the Author

Dr. Usman is an MD, now pursuing his post-graduation degree. As a medical doctor, he has deep insight in all aspects of health, fitness and nutrition.

He is a certified nutritionist and a personal trainer. With these qualifications, he has helped countless people reach their health, fitness and weight loss goals.

Dr. Usman is an avid researcher with 20+ publications in internationally accepted peer reviewed journals.

He is an accomplished writer with more than 5 years of writing experience. In this time, he has produced countless blogs, articles and research work on topics related to health, fitness and nutrition.

He is a published author with more than 100+ books published and several more in the pipe line.

Finally, he runs his own blog and posts health, fitness and nutrition related articles there regularly. You can visit his blog at http://hcures.com/

Check out some of the other JD-Biz Publishing books

[Gardening Series on Amazon]

Download Free Books!

http://MendonCottageBooks.com

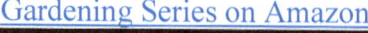

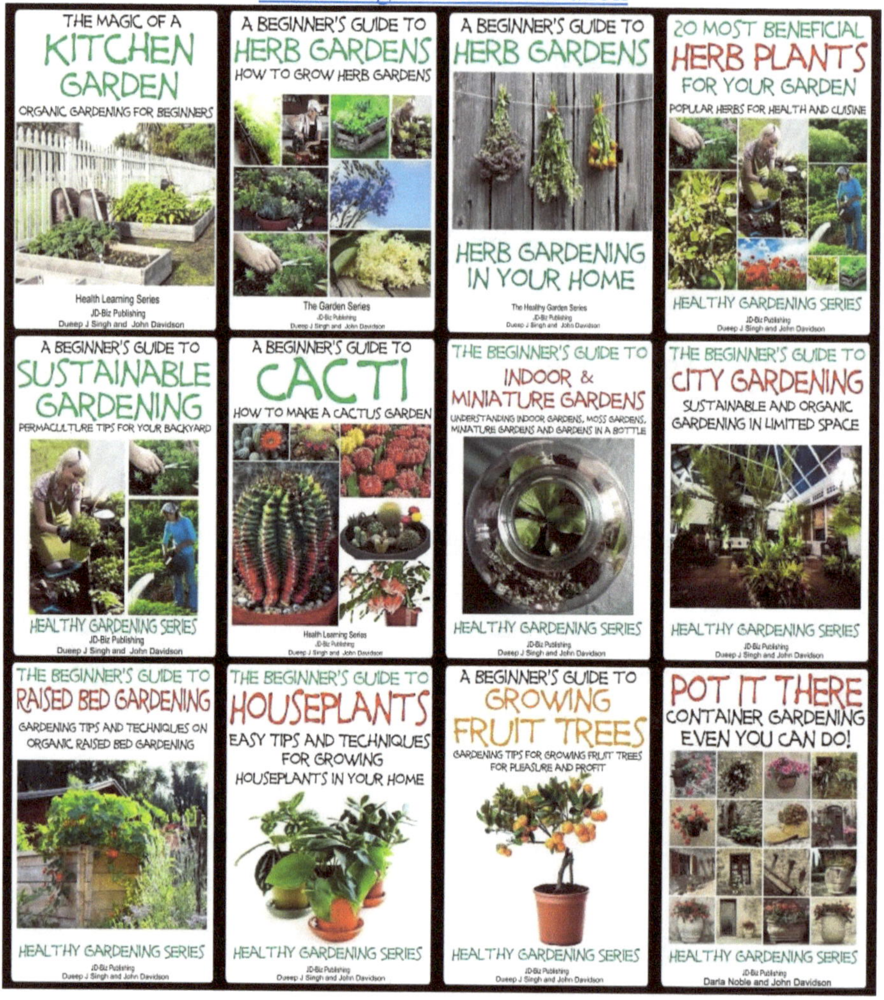

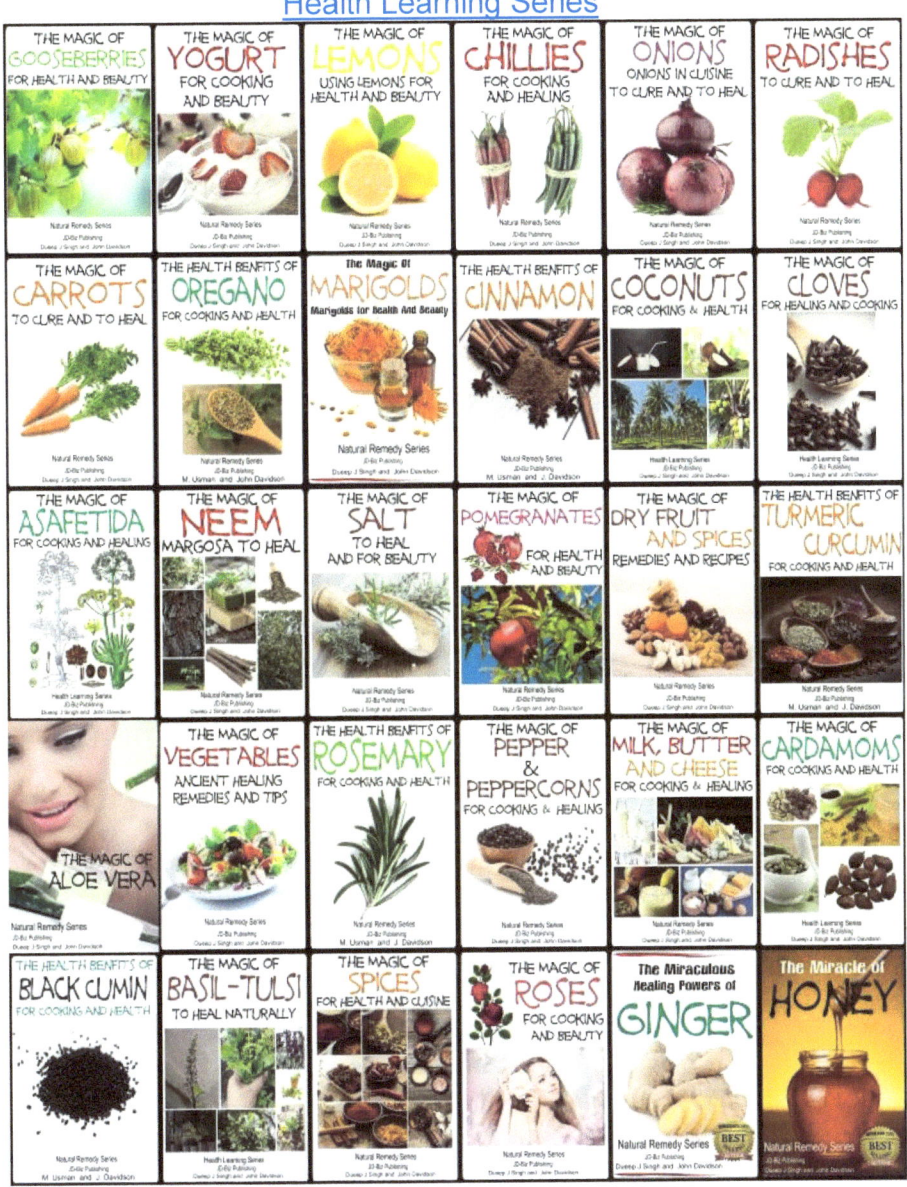

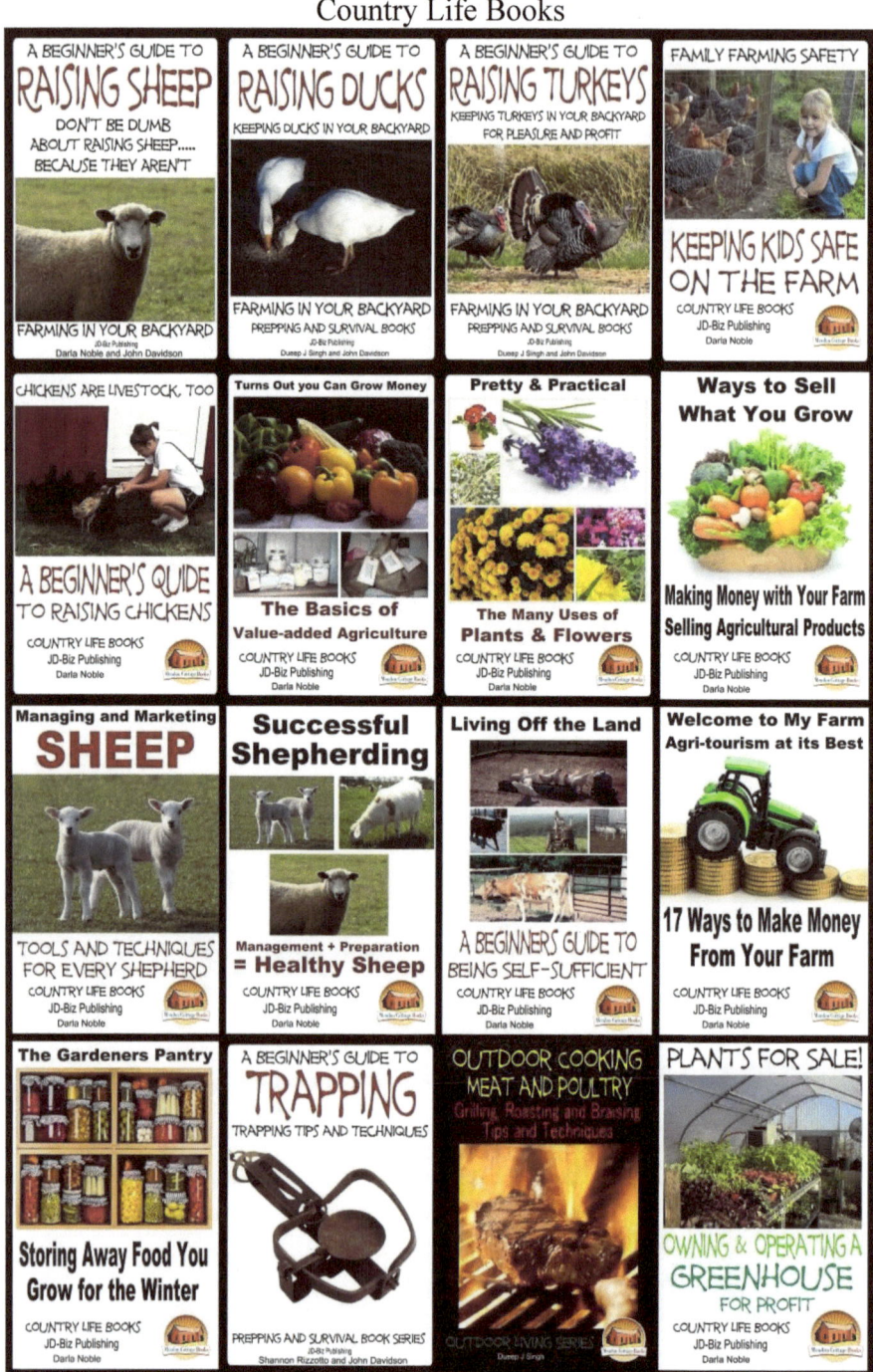

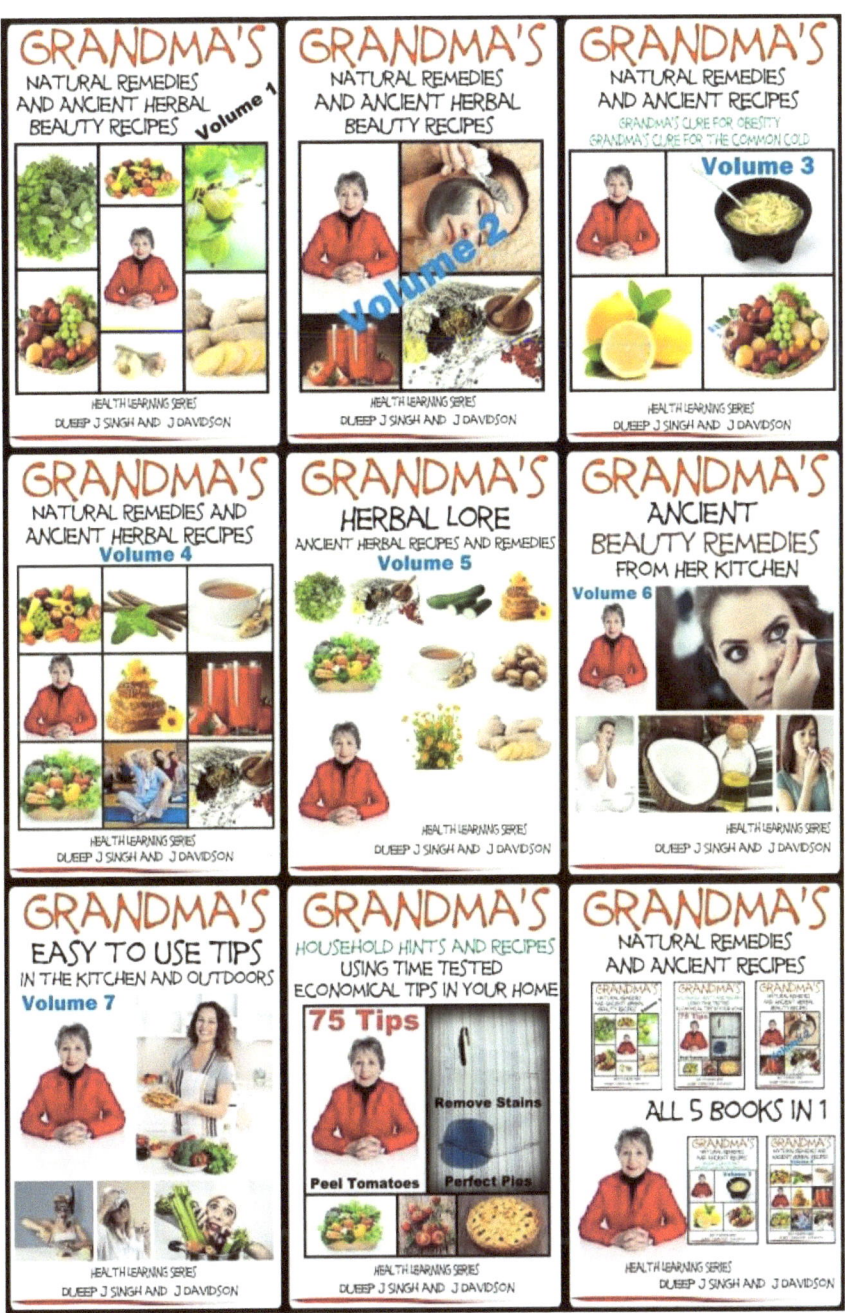

Health Learning Series

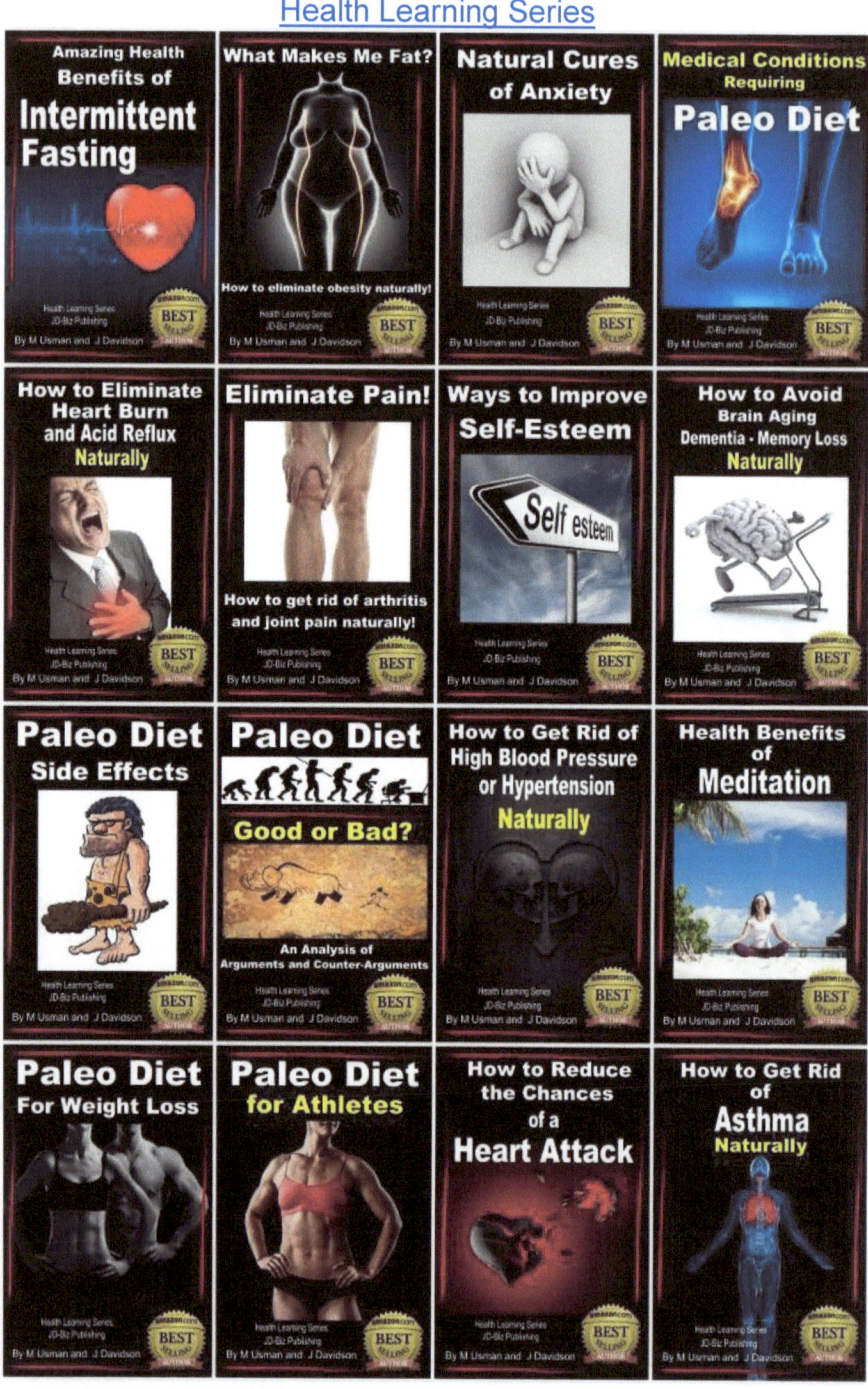

Amazing Animal Book Series

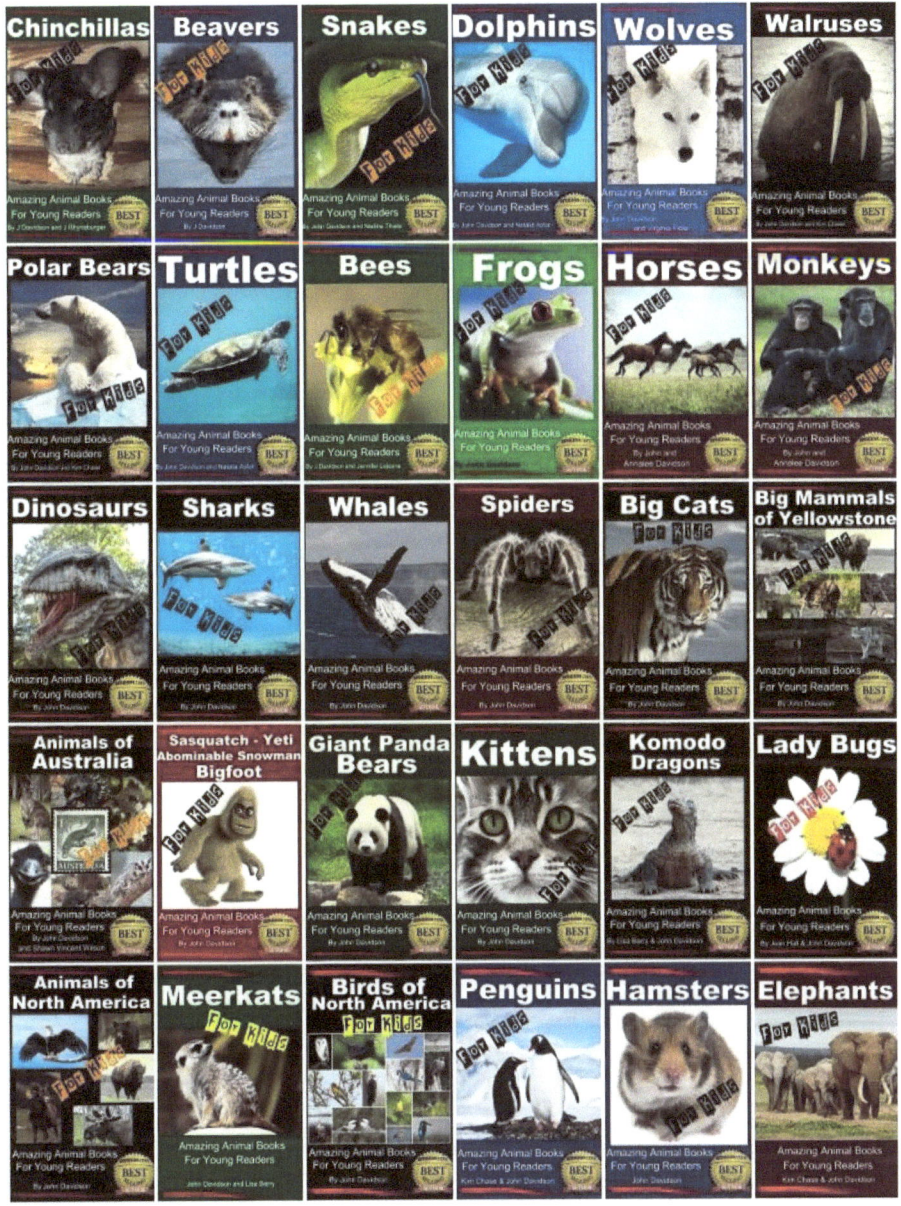

Learn To Draw Series

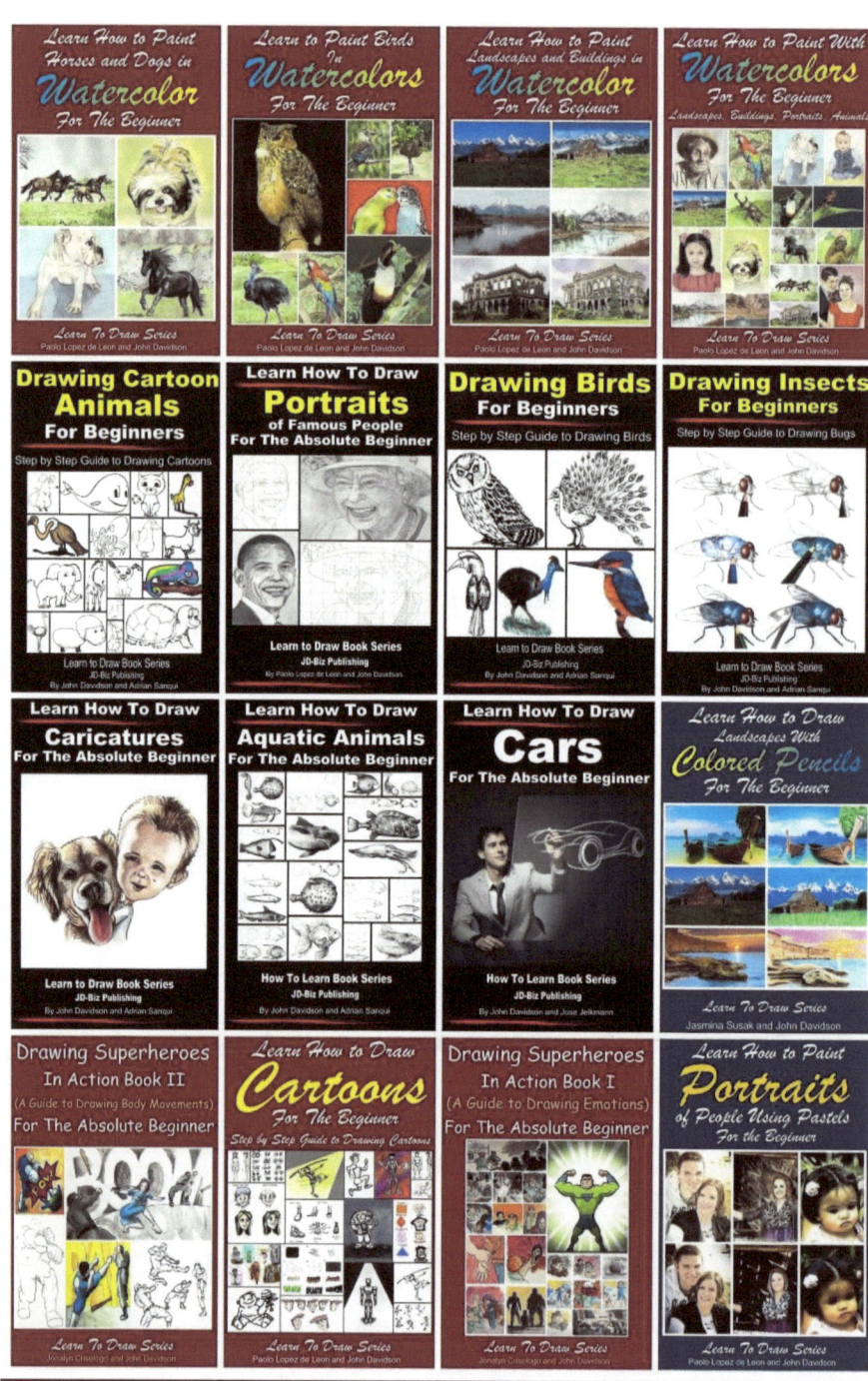

How to Build and Plan Books

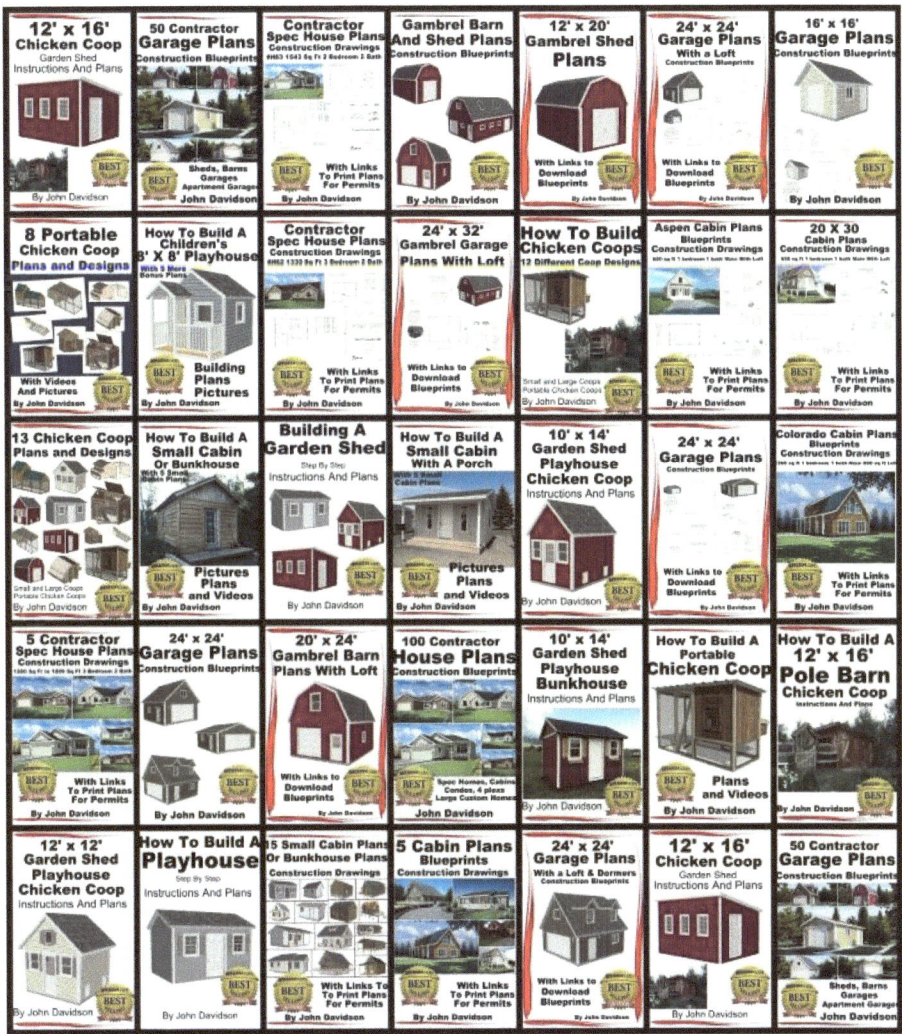

Entrepreneur Book Series

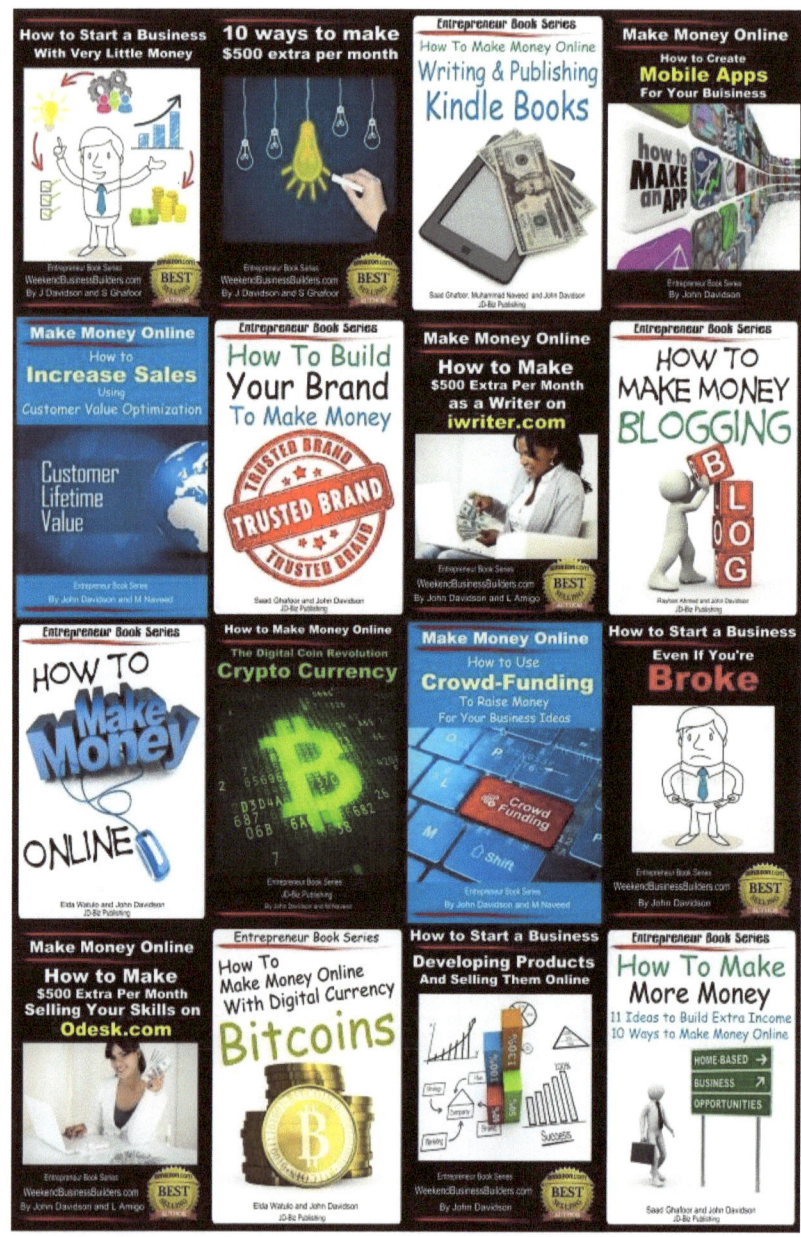

Our books are available at

1. Amazon.com
2. Barnes and Noble
3. Itunes
4. Kobo
5. Smashwords
6. Google Play Books

Download Free Books!

http://MendonCottageBooks.com

Publisher

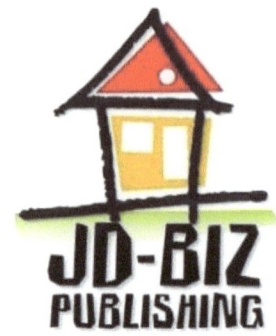

JD-Biz Corp

P O Box 374

Mendon, Utah 84325

http://www.jd-biz.com/

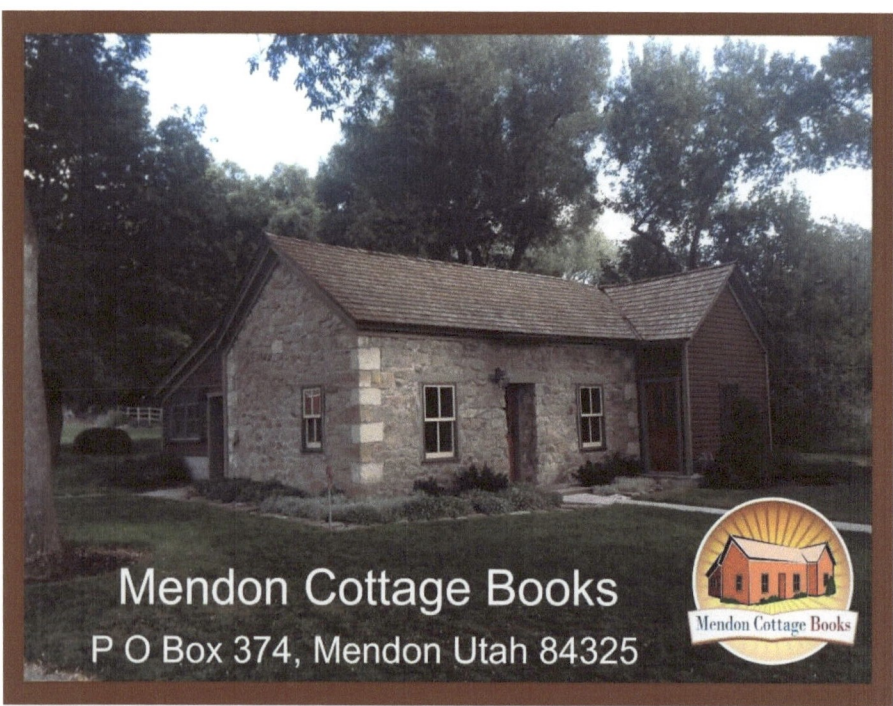

Mendon Cottage Books

P O Box 374, Mendon Utah 84325

www.ingramcontent.com/pod-product-compliance
Lightning Source LLC
Chambersburg PA
CBHW050833290526
45792CB00001B/369